Freque

all about
DHEA

RAY SAHELIAN, MD

AVERY PUBLISHING GROUP
Garden City Park • New York

The information contained in this book is based upon the research and personal and professional experiences of the author. They are not intended as a substitute for consulting with your physician or other health care provider. Any attempt to diagnose and treat an illness should be done under the direction of a health care professional.

The publisher does not advocate the use of any particular health care protocol, but believes the information in this book should be available to the public. The publisher and author are not responsible for any adverse effects or consequences resulting from the use of any of the suggestions, preparations, or procedures discussed in this book. Should the reader have any questions concerning the appropriateness of any procedure or preparation mentioned, the author and the publisher strongly suggest consulting a professional health care advisor.

ISBN: 0-89529-888-0

Printed in the United States of America

10   9   8   7   6   5   4   3   2   1

Contents

Introduction, 5

1. The ABCs of DHEA, 7

2. DHEA and Aging, 15

3. DHEA and the Brain, 21

4. DHEA and the Heart, 27

5. Cancer Control, 33

6. The Immune System, 37

7. Autoimmune Conditions, 43

8. DHEA's Other Effects, 49

9. The Right Dose, 53

10. Cautions and Side Effects, 67

Conclusion, 75

Glossary, 77

References, 81

Suggested Readings, 85

Index, 87

Introduction

Ever since dehydroepiandrosterone (DHEA) became available without a prescription in 1995, its popularity has soared. Countless articles have appeared touting its anti-aging and disease-resisting benefits. At the same time, some physicians and researchers have urged caution with DHEA. It is not surprising that many people have become confused about the benefits and risks of DHEA supplementation.

As is the case with many natural substances, DHEA offers tremendous potential for maintaining health and reversing disease, as well as carrying some risks. While DHEA has benefited many people, some have complained about side effects. Like any supplemental hormone, it should be used under the guidance of a health care professional.

Why has all this attention been lavished on DHEA? Over the past three decades, scientists have examined the role of DHEA in relation to:

- aging

- mental function including mood, memory, and sex drive
- cardiovascular function and cholesterol levels
- immune function
- autoimmune disorders such as lupus
- cancer
- osteoporosis
- obesity
- muscle mass

As a physician, I've examined hundreds of articles on DHEA from the 1950s to the very latest research, interviewed prominent researchers and physicians who are familiar with this hormone, and supervised individuals who are currently using it. My goal in *All About DHEA* is to provide you with a balanced discussion of DHEA. I describe its benefits, its uncertainties, and its shortcomings. I will provide you with the latest information, and then it will be up to you, in consultation with your health care professional, to decide whether DHEA is appropriate for you.

1.

The ABCs of DHEA

There are quite a number of nutrients currently sold in vitamin stores and many of them have complicated names or abbreviations. For example, a quick scan in a health food store will reveal products called NADH, SAM, ALC, PS, and DMAE. You will also find a product that says DHA. DHA stands for *docosahexanoic* acid, which is one of the fatty acids found in fish oils. DHEA (dehydroepiandrosterone) has no relation to DHA. The field of nutritional therapy is getting complicated, and this book will provide you with the answers you need in order to understand the important hormone DHEA.

Q. What is DHEA?

A. DHEA is short for dehydroepiandrosterone, a hormone made mostly by the adrenal glands, but also made in other parts of the body including the testicles, ovaries, and brain. After production in the adrenal glands, DHEA travels in the bloodstream and enters tissues and cells where it is converted into androgens (such as testosterone) and estrogens. Many of these terms are defined in the Glossary at the back of this book.

Q. How is DHEA made in the body?

A. In addition to DHEA, the adrenal glands make a variety of hormones, all starting from cholesterol. Cholesterol is the starting point for all of the steroid hormones. Cholesterol is converted into pregnenolone (another hormone sold over the counter) and then to DHEA, and a number of sex hormones such as testosterone and estrogens. Adrenal hormones play many important roles in the body and have an influence on practically every organ and tissue.

Q. What is a steroid?

A. Steroids are hormones. All of the steroid hormones are made from cholesterol. Some of the steroid hormones include estrogen (the "female hormone"), DHEA, pregnenolone, progesterone (another "female hormone"), and testosterone (the principal "male hormone").

Q. Where does the DHEA sold in stores come from?

A. Vitamin and pharmaceutical companies make the DHEA pills that you buy. They extract sterols (a class of plant hormones) from wild yams, which are grown commercially. The most common sterol is diosgenin, which has a chemical structure similar to the adrenal hormones. DHEA is made by modifying diosgenin molecules in the laboratory.

Q. Will natural yam extract pills increase my DHEA levels?

A. Extracts of wild yams, such as diosgenin, are sold as pills or in a cream. There have been claims that these yam extracts can be converted into DHEA, progesterone, and other hormones by the body. However, the body does not have the necessary enzymes to make these conversions.

Q. How much DHEA do our bodies make?

A. Researchers estimate that humans make between 10 and 15 mg of DHEA daily, although some scientists have estimated higher levels.

Q. Will taking DHEA supplements suppress my natural DHEA production?

A. The production of most steroids is controlled by a "feedback loop." This means that when hormone levels get too high, the body makes less; and when hormone levels are too low, the body makes more. Cortisol, testosterone, and estrogen are all regulated by feedback loops. In other words, if you take cortisol, or a similar derivative such as prednisone, it will shut off your body's natural production of cortisol.

DHEA is an exception to this rule. Preliminary studies do not seem to indicate a feedback mechanism exists for this hormone. In other words, supplements in small dosages will not stop our bodies' own production. However, it's possible that high dosages for prolonged periods could have an influence.

Q. What is DHEAS?

A. DHEA circulates in the bloodstream attached to a mineral called sulfur. The sulfur itself is attached to a few oxygen atoms and hence is called sulfate. Thus DHEAS stands for DHEA-sulfate. DHEA, together with DHEAS, is the most abundant steroid in the blood of young adult humans.

Your body makes most of its DHEA in the morning hours. Its levels decline fairly rapidly during the day because it is quickly cleared by the kidneys. However, DHEAS is cleared slower, and blood levels remain much more stable throughout the day. When researchers want to assess blood levels for DHEA, they generally measure DHEAS levels. When you take DHEA supplements, some of it will circulate in your bloodstream as DHEA, but the majority—90 percent or more—will be combined with sulfur to circulate as DHEAS.

Q. Does DHEA raise levels of other hormones?

A. Yes, it does. For example, numerous studies have found that DHEA administration increases levels of sex hormones, such as estrogen and testosterone. In a recent study done at the Department of Obstetrics and Gynecology, at the University of Pisa in Italy, 100 mg a day of DHEA was given to six postmenopausal women for seven days. A significant increase occurred in circulating levels of androstenedione, testosterone, and estrogens. Androstenedione is a hormone intermediary between DHEA and the sex hormones.

Q. Can DHEA influence the aging process?

A. While aging is inevitable—all living things eventually grow old—the speed of aging varies among animals and people. Some people live to 90 and remain alert and functional. Others, unfortunately, deteriorate and die at much younger ages. The differences in the rate of aging are influenced by many different factors, including heredity, diet, and lifestyle. If you inherit good genes and eat good foods (and avoid junk foods), you improve your odds of living a long and healthy life.

In recent years, scientists have studied some of the biological details of why and how people age. In the process, they have discovered that many beneficial compounds slow the rate of aging and appear to reverse many degenerative diseases. For example, vitamins improve the efficiency of the body and protect it from damaging compounds. In doing so, they slow the aging process. Some vitamins, such as vitamin E, also reduce the risk of heart disease. Since heart disease is largely a disease of aging, vitamin E slows the aging process by slowing the development of disease.

DHEA is similar, though it is not a vitamin. It is a hormone produced by the body, but it is produced in smaller amounts as you get older. Some studies have found that DHEA supplements can reenergize older folks and reverse some diseases. It's not quite a fountain of youth, but it appears to make many older people feel younger. Taking DHEA is similar to women taking estrogen-replacement therapy to look and feel younger, except that DHEA can have a positive and invigorating effect on both sexes. But like estrogen, it has to be taken judiciously and, ideally, under the guidance of a physician.

Q. Is it okay if I self-medicate with DHEA?

A. I recommend that you see a health care practitioner who is familiar with its use before you use it. Although DHEA is available without a prescription, it is not completely free of risks—but then, nothing is. I will discuss the side effects and cautions related to DHEA later in this book.

2.

DHEA and Aging

When DHEA first became popular, there were many articles and books published on this hormone claiming it could reverse the aging process. Many articles were also published in medical journals with both pro and con opinions on DHEA. The attention focused on DHEA in the United States even reverberated throughout the world with numerous editorials written in foreign journals. In this chapter, we look at DHEA and how it is involved in the aging process.

Q. What happens to the body's production of DHEA with age?

A. Although a fetus makes DHEA, and this hormone is present in a baby for the first few months of life, there is very little made from six months up to the beginnings of puberty. From then on, DHEA levels continually rise and peak when we are in our 20s. From our 30s on, there is a progressive decline in DHEA levels. Researchers estimate that by age 70 we only make a fourth of the amounts made in our prime, and by age 90, perhaps a tenth. Levels in women are generally lower, and there is a sharper decline in women after menopause since the ovaries also make DHEA. Furthermore, there are occasionally healthy older individuals who have higher blood levels of this steroid than some younger individuals. DHEA levels decline not only with age but also during certain types of illness or stress.

Q. Do all hormones decline with age?

A. Not all of the hormones produced in our bodies decline with age the way that DHEA does. Estrogen, made by the ovaries, declines sharply only after menopause. Melatonin, made by the pineal gland, declines progressively as the decades march on. However, other hormones made by the adrenal glands, such as cortisol and aldosterone, stay relatively stable throughout life. Levels of insulin, made by the pancreas, and thyroid hormone, can vary depending on a person's medical condition.

Q. What are the potential benefits of hormone supplementation?

A. A number of physiological changes occur in our bodies as we age. For instance, there's a substantial reduction in protein synthesis leading to shrinkage in muscle mass, as well as decreased bone formation leading to osteoporosis. These changes are partly related to the age-associated decline in hormones. Many "anti-aging" physicians believe that restoring these declining hormones can:

- slow the progression of aging
- preserve mental function
- maintain a healthy heart
- delay muscle wasting
- strengthen bones
- improve immune function

Although hormones have very important functions in the body, it would be naïve to expect them to magically reverse many aspects of the aging process. However, preliminary research indicates that the replacement of some hormones could have a positive influence on many biological processes in the body. For example, it is well accepted that estrogen replacement in postmenopausal women can reduce the risk of osteoporosis and heart disease. Estrogen replacement can also increase the risk of endometrial cancer and possibly also breast cancer. Hence, the whole issue of hormone replacement is still a hotly debated one and there is no consensus among doctors on which hormones, if any, should be replaced, and in what combinations, forms, and dosages. I will provide some specific guidelines on hormone replacement with DHEA and other hormones later in this book.

Q. Have there been long-term studies with DHEA in aging people?

A. Several DHEA studies, lasting six months or longer, have been conducted on humans. In one of the studies, Samuel Yen, M.D., and his colleagues at the University of San Diego in La Jolla, California, gave 100 mg of DHEA to eight men and eight women, ages of 50 and 65, for six months. This is a pretty high dose, and blood levels of DHEAS increased several-fold in the subjects. The androgen levels doubled in the men, and quadrupled in the women. One of the eight women developed facial hair. Lean body mass increased in both men and women, there was some increase in muscle strength of the knee. No changes occurred in lipid profiles, insulin or glucose levels, nitrogen balance, bone mineral density, or basal metabolic rate.

Q. Can you tell me about other human research on DHEA as we age?

A. Researchers at Center Hospital University of Laval, Quebec, Canada, gave DHEA for twelve months to fifteen postmenopausal women, ages of 60 and 70. The DHEA was in the form of a cream applied to the inner thighs. The blood DHEAS levels were monitored monthly and the dose of the DHEA was adjusted to sustain levels of DHEAS in their blood similar to those of young people between the ages of 20 and 30. At the conclusion of the study, 80 percent of the women had a greater feeling of well being. There was no change in body weight, but a 10-percent decrease in body fat was replaced by a 10-percent increase in muscle mass. Blood sugar and insulin levels decreased slightly, suggesting greater resistance to diabetes. Cholesterol levels decreased minimally, as did all lipoprotein fractions including LDL (the so-called bad cholesterol) and HDL (the so-called good cholesterol). The HDL/cholesterol ratios did not change, and triglyceride levels did not change.

In addition, the researchers reported that sebum (oil) secretion in skin increased by 70 percent, and vaginal epithelium showed more maturation (meaning that DHEA had a beneficial estrogenic effect on vaginal tissue). These changes are typical of a younger body. Uterine lining did not show stimulation, which is good, because estrogen overstimulates uterine tissue and leads to a higher risk of uterine cancer. There was also a significant increase in bone density. However, the researchers did not evaluate scalp hair, breast tissue, or immune function. During my interview with Dr. Diamond, he mentioned that some of the women had acne and increased libido. In a sense, they developed some of the characteristics of teenagers.

3.

DHEA and the Brain

Scientists now believe that mood, personality, behavior, and thoughts, are, to a large extent, influenced by brain chemicals called *neurotransmitters* (a chemical in the brain that allows signals to be transferred from one brain cell to the next). There are at least sixty neurotransmitters in our central nervous system that have been identified so far, and undoubtedly more will be discovered in the future.

Q. Is DHEA found in the brain?

A. The adrenal glands make at least 150 different steroid compounds, including pregnenolone and DHEA. In the past, some of these metabolites were thought to be inactive. However, we now know that they have a role in influencing behavior and memory. They can act on many receptors in the brain, including serotonin. Some of the cells of the human brain have the ability to synthesize DHEA. Therefore, DHEA can be considered to be a neurohormone, (any hormone found in the brain).

Q. Do brain DHEA levels decline or change with age?

A. Just as blood levels of DHEA decline with age, brain levels of DHEA also decline with age. Dr. Guazzo and colleagues, from the University of Cambridge, England, have discovered that levels of DHEA in cerebrospinal fluid—the fluid that bathes the brain and spinal cord—also decline with age. Interestingly, the ratio of cortisol (a "stress" hormone) to DHEA was found to increase with age. This means that with age, there was less DHEA in the brain relative to cortisol. The researchers state, "These changes may have important implications for age-related alterations in brain function."

Q. Would supplementing with DHEA as we get older improve brain function?

A. Estrogen replacement has been found to improve certain aspects of mental functioning and to perhaps decrease the incidence of Alzheimer's disease. It's quite possible that as more scientific information becomes available, we may discover that replacing other steroid hormones, such as pregnenolone and DHEA, would also benefit cognition.

Q. Does DHEA influence mood?

A. It can—often in a good way, sometimes in a negative way. Consider a study by Dr. Owen Wolkowitz of the Department of Psychiatry, University of California, San Francisco. He gave six depressed middle-aged and elderly individuals about 30 mg of DHEA for one month. Blood tests for DHEA were monitored to reach levels found normally in younger people. At the conclusion of the study, the patients had a significant improvement in memory and mood. When I talked with Dr. Wolkowitz, he told me, "Our research has consistently shown that DHEA supplementation improves mood."

In addition, other studies have also found that DHEA increases energy levels and a sense of well being in a majority of users, and I have found this in my clinical experience as well. However, some people complain of greater irritability and overstimulation with DHEA, particularly if very high doses are taken.

Q. Does DHEA affect memory?

A. Although no formal studies have been done specifically examining the role of DHEA replacement and memory in humans, many patients report feeling more alert and having a clarity of thinking while taking this hormone.

Evidence from animal studies shows that DHEA may aid memory in rodents. While it is not yet known whether this translates to human benefit, the studies are encouraging. In 1992, Dr. James Flood of the St. Louis University School of Medicine, gave DHEA, pregnenolone, and other steroid hormones to a group of mice and found the hormone to test their influence on memory. Mice were placed in a T-shaped maze and given 5 seconds after a bell sounded to find their way into the correct arm of the T. If they failed to do so within 5 seconds, they were electrically shocked until they succeeded. Once trained in the procedure, the mice were injected with a steroid hormone or a placebo. One week later, they were retested for retention of the learned response.

While many steroids were found to reduce the number of runs required for the mice to relearn the shock-avoidance procedure, DHEA was effective. The dosage ranges over which different steroids enhanced memory and learning in these mice was unusual. Most steroid hormones were found to enhance learning only within a two- to five-fold dose range. These observations suggest that DHEA plays a special role in the brain.

Q. Does DHEA protect against brain-cell damage?

A. Researchers at the Department of Anatomy, University of Cambridge, England, have found that DHEA can prevent or reduce the toxic actions in the hippocampus (an area in the brain involved in memory) when exposed to glutamate compounds. The release of glutamate, an amino acid, in the brain after strokes has been implicated in neural damage. The researchers stated, "Our results suggest that decreased DHEA levels may contribute significantly to the increased vulnerability of the aging or stressed human brain to such damage."

Similar benefits with DHEA have been observed by researchers in the Department of Anatomy, University of Arkansas, Little Rock. Laboratory research on isolated brain cells has determined DHEA to protect against brain cell damage. The researchers say, "Levels of DHEA and its sulfated derivative DHEA-S decline during aging and reach even lower levels in Alzheimer's disease. Our findings imply that age-related declines in the availability of DHEA-S could exacerbate neurotoxicity."

4.

DHEA and the Heart

Heart disease is the leading cause of death in the United States. The known ways we can improve our heart health are by consuming a diet high in fiber, low in saturated fat, adequate in mono/polyunsaturated/fish oils, high in dietary antioxidants complete with a variety of fresh fruits and vegetables, and to get plenty of exercise. You are probably familiar with this advice. Recent studies have reviewed the association between heart disease and DHEA levels, and the role DHEA plays as a blood thinner and as a possible antioxidant.

Q. Is DHEA associated with a lower risk of heart disease?

A. Results from one study showed a lower risk of heart disease in men with high levels of DHEAS. In

1998, researchers at the New England Research Institute, Watertown, Massachusetts, analyzed data from the Massachusetts Male Aging Study (MMAS). This provided a large population-based random sample of 1,709 men, 40 to 70 years of age, in which to examine the relation of DHEA and DHEAS levels to heart disease.

The researchers concluded, "Serum concentrations of the adrenal androgen dehydroepiandrosterone (DHEA) and its sulfate ester (DHEAS), both of which decline with age more markedly than other sex hormone levels, have been alternately credited and discredited as 'protective' correlates of heart disease. These findings suggest that serum DHEAS levels bear an inverse relationship to heart disease, independently of a large set of established cardiovascular risk factors." While promising, this study showed a relationship between high DHEA levels and low risk of heart disease. This is not the same as showing cause and effect.

Q. What are "blood thinners"?

A. Anti-clotting agents, or blood thinners, are often recommended or prescribed to patients who have had heart attacks or to those at risk of heart disease. One of the major causes of heart attacks is a clot that forms in the coronary arteries, reducing or stopping blood flow to a major section of the heart muscle. Therefore, medicines that are blood thinners are often recommended in the hope of preventing the clots from occurring. Aspirin is an example of a blood thinner that many people know about, although high dosages can lead to excess bleeding.

Q. Is DHEA a blood thinner?

A. While DHEA has not been shown to be a blood thinner, it has been shown to slow the platelet aggregation that causes clotting. In one study, researchers at the Medical College of Virginia, Richmond, gave DHEA to five healthy young men three times daily for fourteen days and then tested their platelets. The results were compared to another five men who received placebo pills. Four out of the five men on DHEA had their platelet aggregation rates prolonged. In other words, it took their blood longer to clot. This anti-platelet activity could be beneficial in patients who are prone to heart attacks.

Q. Is DHEA an antioxidant?

A. Many people are now familiar with antioxidants—substances that protect our cells from free-radical damage that can lead to cancer—such as vitamins E and C. Recent studies have shown that DHEA also has antioxidant properties that may reduce the risk of heart disease.

Canadian researchers at the Centre de Recherche en Gerontologie, Institut Universitaire de Geriatrie, Sherbrooke, Quebec, evaluated the role of DHEA in protecting the low-density lipoprotein form of cholesterol, known as LDL. Oxidized (damaged) LDL in the blood is believed to play a central role in the events that initiate atherosclerosis, or hardening of the arteries. Antioxidants have been shown to decrease the oxidation of LDLs, leading to the reduction of atherosclerosis. LDLs were obtained from ten healthy subjects and oxidized by free radicals. It was found that DHEA was able to inhibit the oxidation of LDLs by reducing over 90 percent of the free radicals, as well as by reducing the vitamin E loss.

Q. Can high doses of DHEA *cause* a heart risk?

A. Some people have had bad reactions from taking high doses of this hormone. The most serious side effects have related to heart irregularities.

Having mentioned some of the potential positive

benefits of DHEA, you should not assume that the more you take of this hormone the healthier you will be. A small amount of DHEA may be fine, but a larger amount can cause minor or serious side effects. The mechanism for DHEA causing these disturbances is not clear, but could involve a direct action on the rhythm conduction system of the heart.

5.

Cancer Control

As we all know, genetics, smoking, and diet play some of the key roles in the initiation and progression of cancerous tumors. Smoking is certainly related to lung cancer; diet is believed to influence breast, colon, and prostate cancers; and genetics has the strongest influence on childhood cancers. Since the focus of this book is on DHEA, the main question to examine is how are steroids involved in cancer? This issue is very complicated and studies thus far have not been consistent. Even after evaluating estrogen replacement therapy for over four decades we still don't have clear answers.

Q. In general, what do the studies indicate about DHEA and cancer?

A. It's very difficult and expensive to do long-term

studies in humans. It's much easier to do the studies in rodents, but extrapolating these results to humans can sometimes give us false leads. The majority of the research done on mice and rats has shown that DHEA inhibits the development of experimental tumors of the breast, lung, colon, skin, and lymphatic and other tissue. A recent study has again confirmed that DHEA can prevent breast tumors in rodents. Even though a large number of these animal studies have shown DHEA to protect against cancer, the use of hormones in people may yield very different responses. This is especially true of DHEA since very little of this steroid is found in the bloodstream of rodents.

Q. How does DHEA affect prostate cancer?

A. Ever since the introduction of DHEA into the marketplace, a debate has raged as to whether it is a beneficial hormone for those who have prostate cancer, or whether it can be a detriment. A number of animal studies have indicated that DHEA has potent anti-tumor abilities. It has also been proposed that DHEA, being a weak androgen, could potentially attach to the available receptors in prostate tissue and prevent the influence of more potent androgens, which could cause the prostate gland to enlarge. On the other hand, since DHEA can convert into testosterone and dihydrotestosterone, hormones that are believed to stimulate prostate tissue, it has also been proposed that DHEA can stimulate the growth of the prostate gland, which can lead to cancer.

One particular case study, published in the journal *Urology*, sheds light on this issue. A patient with advanced prostate cancer was treated with DHEA after other treatment regimens (such as chemotherapy) failed. Many of his symptoms and signs, including anemia (low blood count), improved on DHEA therapy. However, there was a flare-up of his prostate cancer. This flare-up was controlled with *anti*-hormone therapy.

The dose of DHEA prescribed to this patient was very high—about 140 times more than I usually recommend. DHEA, even though it is available over the counter, has profound effects on the body and, as I've mentioned before, should always be used in low dosages.

Q. Is it possible to safely administer DHEA for prostate cancer?

A. It is possible that administering a medicine

that blocks the conversion of testosterone to dihydrotestosterone along with DHEA could potentially be beneficial in decreasing, or minimizing the side effects of DHEA. Such a medicine does exist, and it's called finasteride, but proper testing has not been done yet to determine whether this hypothesis is correct.

Q. Would you recommend caution in using DHEA as a cancer treatment?

A. Due to the evidence thus far collected, I would recommend using caution in using DHEA to help cancer treatment. Too little is known about the role of supplemental DHEA in initiating, preventing, or treating cancer in humans. Unfortunately, the longest double-blind, well-controlled, published studies of DHEA administration to humans have only been twelve months. Since cancer cells often take many months and years to grow into obvious tumors, we haven't had enough time to study the role of DHEA supplements in human cancers. The best we can do is make an intelligent prediction based on the available laboratory and animal data, and also based on our present understanding of the physiological role of DHEA and its metabolites.

6.

The Immune System

After heart disease, cancer, and stroke, the other leading causes of death in the US are due to infections. As we go on in years, our immune systems don't work as well as they should. Since DHEA(S) levels decline with age, and due to promising results in animal studies, it has been suggested that supplementation in older individuals could improve certain functions of the immune system.

Q. What exactly is the immune system?

A. The immune system is the body's defense mechanism to neutralize or destroy undesirable invaders such as infections, viruses, or allergens.

The immune system is made up of many cells that have various functions. There are many types of immune cells traveling in your bloodstream. You

have heard of white blood cells. Lymphocytes are a
type of white blood cell that have multiple functions, including forming antibodies to fight off
germs, and being constantly on the lookout for any
cells in our bodies that could be turning cancerous.
When these abnormal cells start growing, our lymphocytes go on a search and destroy mission. Two
major types of lymphocytes are T cells and B cells.
Natural killer cells and macrophages are other cells
that are part of the immune system.

The immune system also produces a number of
substances that are involved in keeping us germ-
free. Some of the names you have heard of before,
such as antibodies and interferon, others may be
new to you, such as lymphokines. In order for a
hormone to influence immune cells more effective-
ly, it is important that there be sites on the cell
where it can attach. These areas are called receptors.
Researchers from Kyushu University in Fukuoka,
Japan have found receptors (docking bays, so to
speak) for DHEA on our T cells.

Q. Does DHEA improve how the immune system works?

A. It seems to. Nine healthy elderly men with an
average age of 64 years took 50 mg of DHEA night-

ly for twenty weeks. DHEA treatment significantly elevated natural killer cells. Although the number of T lymphocytes was unaffected, T cell function was increased, and B cell function was also increased.

Q. How does AIDS affect the immune system?

A. After an individual is infected with HIV (human immunodeficiency virus), there is usually a period of gradual immune decline eventually reaching a stage of very low immune status—making the body highly susceptible to a number of viruses, bacteria, fungi, and parasites. This low immune state is known as AIDS (acquired immune deficiency syndrome). There are multiple factors that are associated with the progression to AIDS, including nutritional deficiencies and diminished resistance to oxidative stress.

T cells are an important part of the immune system. There are a number of T cells, each with a different name and function. HIV usually infects a type of T cell called helper/inducer (also referred to as CD4). As a consequence, the AIDS patient becomes very susceptible to organisms that a healthy immune system fights off very easily. The term "opportunistic infections" is given to these bacteria, viruses, fungi, or parasites. Individuals with normal immune systems will have a CD4 count of over 800 cells per milliliter of blood, whereas HIV infected individuals with opportunistic infections have a count of less than 200.

Q. What is the relationship between AIDS and DHEA levels?

A. In a study at Louisiana State University Medical Center in New Orleans, researchers evaluated the blood levels for cortisol and DHEAS in ninety-eight adults with HIV. There was a significant correlation between DHEAS and CD4 levels, but not between cortisol and CD4 levels. Those who had low DHEAS levels also had low levels of CD4. They concluded, "The data exhibit a positive relationship between the immune status of patients with HIV-related illness and DHEA, leading to the hypothesis that DHEA deficiency may worsen immune status."

We also know that the adrenal cortex of individuals with HIV is commonly infected with the virus. Autopsies done on patients who died from AIDS have shown that in more than half of the cases, the adrenal glands had been infected with an opportunistic fungus, bacterium, or virus. Some even had cancers of the adrenal glands. Over many years of the illness, it would be likely that secretion of DHEAS would be lowered.

Q. If DHEA were given to patients with AIDS would their symptoms improve? Or might DHEA supplementation slow the progression of HIV infection to AIDS?

A. Dr. Dyner and colleagues, at the California Pacific Medical Center in San Francisco, gave 750 mg of DHEA for sixteen weeks to thirty-one HIV infected men with CD4 counts between 250 and 600 cells/ml. There were no improvements in CD4 counts. We do not know whether lower doses of supplemental DHEA may have given different results. Also not known is how DHEA will influence other aspects of the immune system in individuals with AIDS.

DHEA, though, has been found in one small study to inversely correlate with cognitive function in AIDS patients. In six patients with HIV, ages ranging from thirty to fifty-one years, lower DHEAS levels were associated with more cognitive impairment. The researchers conclude, "Our preliminary data encourage further investigation of the relationship between DHEAS levels and HIV-associated cognitive impairment. DHEAS may represent a useful metabolic marker in combination with neurologic and neuropsychologic examination, in the evaluation of HIV-infected individuals with cognitive complaints."

Q. What steps can I take to improve my immune system?

A. There are many ways to improve your immune system. Deep sleep, moderate exercise, variety of fresh fruits and vegetables, low stress, positive attitude, multivitamins and minerals, (especially C, B, and zinc) and certain antioxidants are a few of the accepted ways. Herbs such as echinacea and goldenseal also have their believers. Chronic stress is known to impair the immune system, partly since stress increases the adrenal glands' output of cortisol. Cortisol causes significant immune system depression.

7.

Autoimmune Conditions

There are times when our immune system malfunctions. Two different types of mistakes that can be made are: 1) a foreign organism is not recognized as such and allowed to squat and set up camp, and 2) the body's tissues and cells are mistakenly identified as foreign and are mercilessly attacked. This latter mistake is known as autoimmunity (immunity to self). There are many autoimmune conditions, including systemic lupus erythematosus, pemphigoid and pemphigus, and rheumatoid arthritis. DHEA may be of benefit in normalizing immune function.

Q. What is lupus?

A. Lupus is an inflammatory disease that can cause inflammation of the blood vessels, kidney disorders, and tumors on the skin and within the nervous system. Symptoms include painful and swollen joints, skin rash, and mouth ulcers. Systemic lupus erythematosus (SLE) is four times as common in women than in men. A special blood test, called the antinuclear antibody test, is used for diagnosis.

Q. Does DHEA help patients with lupus?

A. It may. Studies have shown a correlation between low levels of DHEA and lupus.

Dr. Suzuki and colleagues, from St. Marianna University School of Medicine, Kangawa, Japan, have found that nearly all of the patients with SLE that they have examined have had low levels of DHEA. In a test tube, they found providing DHEA to the lymphocytes of the patients restored a powerful immune chemical known as interleukin-2. They conclude, "These results indicate that defects of interleukin-2 synthesis of patients with SLE are at least in part due to the low DHEA activity in the serum."

Dr. van Vollenhoven and colleagues at the Division of Immunology and Rheumatology, Stanford University Medical Center, California, recently published a study reporting their findings of DHEA therapy in lupus. In an uncontrolled longitudinal study, fifty female patients (thirty-seven pre-menopausal and thirteen postmenopausal) with mild to moderate SLE were treated with 50 mg of oral DHEA per day. DHEA therapy was associated with increases in the serum levels of DHEA, DHEAS, and testosterone and, for those patients who continued DHEA, with decreasing disease compared to baseline.

Concurrent prednisone doses were reduced. These improvements were sustained over the entire treatment period. Thirty-four patients (68 percent) completed six months of treatment and twenty-one patients (42 percent) completed twelve months. Acne was the most common adverse event and occurred in over half of the patients. Pre- and post-menopausal women experienced similar efficacy and adverse effects from DHEA. According to the researchers, the hormone appeared clinically beneficial, with the benefits sustained for at least one year in those patients who maintained therapy.

Q. What is rheumatoid arthritis?

A. Rheumatoid arthritis (RA) is a chronic inflammatory disease of unknown origin, with a strong genetic component, that has a tendency to involve joints leading to joint destruction, deformity, and loss of function. RA afflicts about 2 percent of the population, being more common in older women. In addition to joint involvement, patients also often experience fatigue and depression.

Q. Can DHEA help rheumatoid arthritis?

A. While studies are still inconclusive on this issue, DHEA might be worth a try.

Researchers at the University of Bellvitge, Barcelona, Spain, evaluated bone mineral density, levels of testosterone, and DHEAS in a group of ninety-nine men with RA and compared them with another group of men of similar age who did not have this condition. There was reduced bone mineral density in men with RA and also reduced levels of testosterone and DHEAS. Men who had been on corticosteroids also had decreased levels of DHEAS.

Italian researchers measured DHEA levels in ten RA and seven healthy control patients. Average DHEA levels were significantly lower in RA patients than in controls. A trial administering DHEA to individuals with RA has not yet been published.

Q. What are pemphigus and pemphigoid?

A. These are autoimmune skin diseases that lead to blistering on the skin. With pemphigus, the patient loses weight, and becomes weak, and is at risk for infections.

Q. Can DHEA help treat pemphigus and pemphigoid?

A. While studies involving the treatment of these diseases with DHEA supplementation have not yet been conducted, a relationship between the natural levels of DHEA and the occurrence of these diseases has been discovered.

Blood levels of DHEA(S) were measured in twenty-one men and twenty-nine women with these skin problems and compared to twenty patients with psoriasis and twenty-three with osteoarthritis. Psoriasis and osteoarthritis are not autoimmune diseases. The average levels of DHEAS were markedly lower in the pemphigoid/pemphigus group. The researchers concluded, "These low levels are consistent with those reported for SLE, RA and polymyalgia rheumatica/giant cell arteritis. DHEAS deficiency is a permanent feature in these autoimmune diseases, and may contribute to their etiology and/or pathophysiology."

8.

DHEA's Other Effects

Steroid hormones have a profound influence on many important organs and tissues of the body. Hence, in addition to its influence on the brain, immune system, heart, and other systems already discussed, DHEA can also influence muscle, fat cells, skin, hair, and other tissues. Let's examine this hormone's multiple effects.

Q. Can DHEA help me lose weight?

A. While the current evidence points towards helping obesity, DHEA has the interesting effect of increasing muscle tissue and decreasing fat.

In one study, postmenopausal women on DHEA did not lose weight, but there was a 10-percent shift after one year from fat tissue to muscle tissue.

While the human studies have not shown actual weight loss, DHEA has been shown to have anti-obesity activity in dogs. Researchers at the University of Wisconsin, School of Veterinary Medicine, in Madison evaluated the effect of DHEA or placebo combined with a low-fat/high-fiber diet in spontaneously obese dogs. DHEA-treated dogs had a significantly increased rate of actual and percent excess weight loss compared with placebo-treated dogs. The researchers say, "DHEA in combination with caloric restriction results in a faster rate of weight loss than does caloric restriction alone."

Q. Does DHEA influence sex drive?

A. DHEA is converted in the body into testosterone and estrogen. It is known that testosterone increases sexual drive in both men and women. In my clinical experience, many men and women who take DHEA have reported a noticeable increase in sexual interest.

Q. Does DHEA help improve bone density?

A. Researchers from the Rowett Research Institute, Skeletal Research Unit, Bucksburn, Scotland, found that DHEA and DHEAS failed on their own to exert direct, independent significant effects on the growth and differentiation of human osteoblastic (bone-growing) cells. However, treating the cells in conjunction with vitamin D resulted in enhancement of bone growth.

Q. How does DHEA affect skin and hair?

A. Most androgens, such as DHEA, make skin oily. Excess androgens can cause pimples, which is what happens to teenagers. Small dosages are not known to cause acne, except in individuals who are prone to this skin disorder. Large doses of DHEA can cause thinning or loss of scalp hair. Therefore, even though DHEA has many benefits, more is not necessarily better.

Q. Is DHEA use allowed in sports competition?

A. DHEA abuse by athletes has been considered by the International Olympic Committee, which banned the substance in 1998. French scientists at the Laboratoire National de Depistage du Dopage in Chatenay-Malabry, investigated the effect of a single dose of 50 mg of DHEA in healthy men. This hormone was readily absorbed with 50 to 75 percent recovery of dosing in the urine after 24 hours. Conversion of DHEA to the principal biologically active androgen, testosterone, was low but proven to be real.

Q. Is DHEA involved in pregnancy?

A. Venous blood was collected from 151 women at the initiation of labor induction at University of Arizona Health Sciences Center, Department of Obstetrics and Gynecology, Tucson. The average DHEA sulfate level was higher in women who progressed to active labor than in those who did not progress to active labor. The researchers say, "Dehydroepiandrosterone sulfate may be an important factor in successful labor induction." At this point we don't know whether providing DHEA to women near labor will influence the progression to active labor. Women should not use DHEA during labor unless it is recommended by their obstetrician.

9.

The Right Dose

The crucial aspect in supplementing with hormones is finding the right dosage. Unlike some vitamins, such as vitamin C, where a few extra milligrams will make virtually no difference, even one or two mg of DHEA ingested more than required can lead to side effects.

Q. In what forms and in what dosages does DHEA come?

A. Capsules are the most common form, but DHEA also comes in creams, ointments, and even sublingual (beneath the tongue) tablets.

Other forms of DHEA that can be absorbed from the mouth include spray, chewing gum, and liquid. If you buy DHEA without a prescription, you can generally find it in 5, 10, 25, and 50 mg capsules.

Q. Are pills the best form of DHEA to take?

A. One of the practical problems of taking DHEA capsules is that the blood supply from the stomach and intestines goes through the liver before making its way to the rest of the body. The liver is the chemical factory of the body and it makes good sense for it to have "first crack" at the blood supply from the digestive system. Physicians call this the "first-pass effect."

One of the liver's functions is to metabolize sterols and steroids. Cholesterol is a common dietary sterol, and the liver bundles it into lipoproteins (fatty globules) for distribution to body tissues. If there's not enough cholesterol in the foods we eat, the liver makes more of it to make up the difference. The liver also metabolizes DHEA. Because of this, DHEA pills that you swallow may first be metabolized by the liver and the amount that reaches the general circulation will likely be less than the ingested dose. Part of the DHEA may be converted into other androgens like testosterone. The factors that influence absorption from the intestines and metabolism by the liver vary significantly with age and health condition.

Q. What is "micronized" DHEA?

A. One of the ways that pharmacists minimize liver metabolism of steroids is to use "micronized" preparations. Micronization is a process that creates tiny particles that can be absorbed from the intestines into the lymphatic system and somewhat bypass the liver.

Q. What is the best form of DHEA to take?

A. Creams and ointments are acceptable ways to get DHEA into the body. The sublingual, spray, gum, liquid, and micronized versions of DHEA, as well as the creams and ointments, will generally bypass the liver's first-pass effect. Sublingual preparations of many vitamins, drugs, and herbal extracts are common. I believe you should try several forms to see which ones you prefer. Whether, in the long run, avoiding the liver's first-pass effect is healthier and leads to more beneficial outcomes is not known at this time. Since we don't know which form is healthier, I would recommend using the form that provides you with the best clinical response for your particular medical condition. You can also alternate between different forms.

Q. What's the best dosage to start with?

A. I am generally conservative in my approach and prefer most medicines to be started at a low dose. Most of the pills on the market come in 5, 10, 25, and 50 mg. I feel that 5 mg is a good starting dose. If you can only find the higher dosages, you could open the capsules and take a small portion.

Q. What time of day should I take my DHEA?

A. The adrenal gland makes lots of DHEA in the early (pre-dawn) morning, and production drops dramatically throughout the day. I recommend taking DHEA first thing in the morning upon awakening to act in concert with this natural pattern.

Q. Does estrogen replacement interfere with DHEA?

A. Most doctors probably have not considered the effects of estrogen replacement on the levels of other hormones in the body, especially the androgens such as DHEA and testosterone. In a study published by Dr. Casson and colleagues, from the Department of Obstetrics and Gynecology, Baylor College of Medicine, in Houston, Texas, twenty-eight postmenopausal women were given 2 mg a day of oral micronized estradiol for twelve weeks. During this time, levels were measured of various hormones, including DHEA and testosterone. The results of the study showed that estrogen administration lowered blood DHEA levels and also lowered testosterone levels, leading the researchers to conclude that it may be necessary to provide androgen replacement therapy along with estrogen replacement.

Q. Since the hormone pregnenolone can be converted into DHEA, progesterone, and the other steroid hormones, why not use pregnenolone or DHEA exclusively, and let the body convert it into the specific steroid hormones it requires?

A. I think that eventually we'll find that the best hormone replacement regimen involves giving a little bit of pregnenolone, DHEA, and testosterone to men, and pregnenolone, DHEA, and estrogens, and progesterone to women. Young people have the ability to easily convert pregnenolone into all the other steroid hormones. As we age, the enzymes that convert pregnenolone to DHEA, and pregnenolone to progesterone, may not work as well as they once did. Nor would the enzymes that convert DHEA into androgens and estrogens be as effective.

Q. What if you are already on estrogens, could you add DHEA?

A. Since DHEA gets partially converted into female hormones, women would probably need to reduce their dose of estrogens.

Q. Could you provide some general, concise dosage recommendations?

A. The following are some general guidelines on hormone replacement therapy. Please discuss these with your physician if you're planning to take hormones for more than one month. I wish to emphasize that these are suggestions only; in no way do I imply that these dosages are right for everyone. Each of you reading this book has a unique biochemistry. Some of you may not need any of these hormones while others would benefit from higher doses. Also, your health care provider may have a different opinion, believing that the above recommendations are too low, too high, or perhaps inappropriate for you. Listen to your personal physician: He or she knows your medical condition best. (When I refer to hormone holidays, I mean that you go off the hormone two or three days per week, or a week or two per month.

Men: ages 40 to 50: 1 to 4 mg of DHEA in the morning, frequently taking hormone holidays. Or the combination of Preg and DHEA totaling 1 to 4 mg.

Men: ages 50 to 65: 1 to 5 mg of DHEA in the morning, frequently taking hormone holidays, or the combination of Preg and DHEA totaling 1 to 5 mg.

Men: age 65 and older: 2 to 6 mg of DHEA in the morning occasionally taking hormone holidays, or the combination of Preg and DHEA totaling 2 to 6 mg. Supplementing with testosterone is optional, if DHEA by itself does not provide enough of an androgenic effect.

Premenopausal women: age 40 to about 50: 1 to 3 mg of DHEA in the morning, frequently taking hormone holidays, or the combination of Preg and DHEA totaling 1 to 3 mg.

Postmenopausal women, 50 to 65: 1 to 4 mg of DHEA in the morning, occasionally taking hormone holidays, or the combination of Preg and DHEA totaling 1 to 4 mg.

When taking estrogen, you should generally take half the dose normally recommended. For instance, in the case of Premarin, 0.3 mg would be adequate, instead of 0.625. However, I recommend natural or plant estrogens instead of the synthetic versions or those collected from horse urine. Estrogen is available by prescription only. I also recommend you consume between one and four ounces of a soy product a day. This could be in the form of tofu, soy milk, or another form.

If you are taking progesterone, and supplementing with pregnenolone instead of DHEA, or in combination with it, there are special considerations. Since pregnenolone converts into progesterone, the use of pregnenolone makes the need for progesterone less essential. If you do take progesterone, use the natural form in micronized, sublingual, or cream forms. You would need a much lower dose of progesterone if you're already on Preg since some of their effects are similar. Progesterone, in the appropriate strength, is available by prescription.

Women over age 65: 1 to 5 mg of DHEA in the morning, occasionally taking hormone holidays, or the combination of Preg and DHEA totaling 1–5 mg. If you are taking estrogen or progesterone, see the recommendations listed above for Postmenopausal women, 50 to 65.

Q. What about combining hormones and vitamins?

A. I believe in synergism, that is, the use of low doses of many nutrients and hormones instead of a high dose of just one. For instance, instead of taking a high dose of pregnenolone, such as 25 mg, I prefer someone take 1 to 5 mg but, in addition, supplement with other nutrients. Doctors and patients are often looking for the magic pill that, by itself, will cure all ills. The human body is too complicated, with too many biochemical reactions occurring every second, for one pill to be the answer to all problems. The answer lies in intelligently combining a variety of modalities.

Q. How soon will I notice an effect from DHEA?

A. Some users who start with 5 mg will feel an effect that very day. When the dose is raised to 10 mg, more will notice a sense of well-being, often with a sense of heightened alertness and energy. Many individuals also find that DHEA helps increase their interest in sex. Once you notice an effect, you can lower your dosage and take the minimum your body requires. There are individuals who do not feel an effect, even on 50 mg.

Q. What should my doctor and I consider before I take DHEA?

A. The following are some parameters that should be considered while monitoring someone on hormone replacement therapy. These are just guidelines. You may consider having less or more done depending on your particular circumstance. Remember that steroid hormones influence, or are metabolized in, a variety of body tissues including the liver, fat cells, skin, endometrium, myometrium, intestines, breast, kidney, lung, muscle, heart, brain, prostate, testes, ovaries, eyes, and others.

The basics (strongly recommended)
- Weight
- Blood pressure
- Heart rate and rhythm
- Muscle mass

- Body fat
- Eyes
- Hearing
- Skin, particularly for hair growth, moisture, and pimples
- Hair
- Brain function such as mood, alertness, memory, motivation
- Sleep patterns

Additionally in men
- Prostate gland, mostly through finger exam

Additionally in women
- Breast tissue, mostly through palpation, and also possibly through mammograms
- Uterus and cervix, mostly through Pap tests
- Vaginal tissue

Lab tests
- Routine blood panel that includes blood count, white count, kidney function, blood sugar, triglycerides, cholesterol, liver enzymes, and thyroid tests.
- Urinalysis

Q. How important are lab tests for DHEA or DHEA(S) levels?

A. If the above tests are not enough to satisfy your curiosity, you could ask your doctor to do other more extensive, and expensive, testing. My own opinion is that people using DHEA for long periods should only be taking low doses such as 1 to 5 mg, and with breaks. On these low doses, frequent laboratory testing would not be essential; testing two or three times a year may be all that's needed. You can let your own physical signs and symptoms be your guide. Remember that DHEA can accumulate in tissues. Use the lowest effective dose and take "hormone holidays" where you go off it for a few days.

Q. At what age should I get my DHEAS levels tested, and how is it done?

A. Most physicians who incorporate DHEA replacement therapy in their practice will test people starting in their fifties. A blood test is the standard and routine way to check levels, however, it's possible saliva tests can also provide good information. Over the last ten years serum DHEA and DHEA(S) testing services have evolved from obscure research tools to readily available clinical tests. Although a lot of doctors have never ordered tests for DHEA(S) levels, more likely than not the laboratory they use for standard blood tests also does testing for this steroid.

Q. How are DHEA levels measured?

A. When a doctor orders a blood test for you, the results will often come back in micrograms per 100 milliliter (ml) of blood. The laboratory will print on its lab result sheet what the normal ranges are for different age groups. Usually this ranges anywhere from 40 mcg/100 ml which is very low and found in very old people to 400 mcg/100 ml found in young people at their prime. Some labs will also provide the results in nanograms per ml. A nanogram is one thousandth of a microgram.

10.

Cautions and Side Effects

I have interviewed hundreds of individuals who have taken DHEA and there have also been additional studies published on DHEA in the last few years that have provided a better understanding of this hormone's benefits and side effects. Furthermore, our research center has received telephone calls and e-mail messages from DHEA and pregnenolone users informing us of a number of positive and negative reactions.

All this new information prompts me to issue some cautions, which you should take seriously. Until more research is published regarding the long-term safety of DHEA and pregnenolone, I do not recommend you use a regular daily dosage of more than 5 mg unless you are closely monitored by a health care professional familiar with these hormones. I also recommend you take frequent breaks, which I call "hormone holidays." In my opinion, the maximum over-the-counter dosage sold in stores of DHEA and pregnenolone should be no more than 10 mg.

Q. What are some common side effects?

A. Acne and excessive oiliness, facial hair growth in women, irritability, mood changes, overstimulation, and insomnia are among the common side effects. Most of these side effects are dose related and will generally disappear with lower doses of DHEA. Sometimes there will be scalp hair loss or thinning in both women and men. If you experience this problem, stop the DHEA. Your hair should regrow in a few weeks. If you wish to accelerate the regrowth, have your doctor prescribe a medicine called finasteride.

Q. Are there serious side effects from DHEA?

A. Heart irregularities can occur, which are of great concern. Since 1996, I have become aware of at least forty cases of individuals who felt palpitations or irregular heart beats from the use of high-dose

DHEA or the related hormone pregnenolone. I am not certain of how DHEA and pregnenolone cause heart irregularities. Perhaps these hormones have a direct influence on the rhythm-controlling areas of the heart, such as the sinus node or the atrioventricular node, or act indirectly via stimulating the thyroid gland to release more thyroid hormones. Individuals most commonly affected by this problem seem to be the elderly who are already prone to heart irregularities and happen to be taking more than 10 mg of these hormones.

Q. Are there any precautions I can use to protect myself from these side effects, but still benefit from DHEA?

A. If you need to take DHEA or pregnenolone for a particular medical condition, ask your doctor to prescribe a beta-blocker such as propranolol. Carry this medicine with you, and when you feel a palpitation, you can take anywhere between 30 to 60 mg of the propranolol. It should return the heart rate back to normal within a half-hour. Another method that sometimes works is lying down on the floor and elevating the legs, resting them on a wall. Somehow this pools the blood in your body toward your heart, and could return an atrial heart irregularity back to normal sooner. A few individuals have had success with this method. Of course, you can combine both this method and the beta-blocker.

Q. What about DHEA's influence on cancer?

A. Theoretical risks with long-term DHEA supplementation include an influence on hormone-sensitive cancers such as breast, uterine, ovarian, and prostate. High doses of DHEA for prolonged periods could potentially stimulate breast cysts or uterine fibroids. Other theoretical influences with supplementation for many years include positive or negative effects on blood glucose levels, lipids, and other hormones.

Q. Who should not take DHEA?

A. Although we don't know what would happen if pregnant women were given DHEA, we do have an indication that this hormone plays a role in ripening of the cervix. At this time it would be best not to use this hormone during pregnancy or breast feeding unless you are a part of a well-controlled clinical study or your doctor believes it would help you with labor progression. Other individuals who should not take DHEA include those who have excess secretion of androgens, have a susceptibility to androgens, or are on anti-hormone therapy.

Q. Can DHEA be combined with other medicines?

A. A common question that I'm asked is whether other medicines can be taken along with DHEA. Unfortunately, there are hardly any studies published on the combination of DHEA with prescription drugs or supplements. However, based on what is known about DHEA and my knowledge of medicines, I can provide some tentative suggestions.

Antidepressants. Since DHEA can elevate mood and energy in many individuals, the antidepressant dosage required for mood elevation is likely to be less when combined with DHEA. The same applies to St. John's wort, an antidepressant herb. Both the hormone and the antidepressants can act as stimulants, hence, one needs to be careful in stacking these pills.

Estrogen. Because DHEA can convert to estrogens, the dose of estrogen used in hormone replacement therapy may need to be reduced.

Pregnenolone. If you are planning to use both together, the combined dosage should not exceed your planned dosage of one of these hormones. For instance, if you are taking 5 mg of DHEA, and you wish to add pregnenolone, take 3 mg of DHEA and 2 mg of pregnenolone.

Androstenedione. The effects are additive, so follow the recommendations for pregnenolone discussed above.

Aspirin and other blood thinners. DHEA has shown to act as a mild blood thinner, therefore, the dose of other blood thinners may need to be slightly reduced. The herb *Ginkgo biloba*, used as a memory enhancer, also has mild anti-platelet properties.

Stimulants. These include diet pills and even over-the-counter herbs and nutrients, such as ephedra, guarana, caffeine, and others. DHEA is a stimulant itself, and therefore it would not be a good idea to combine high doses of this steroid with other stimulants.

Insulin. There are no apparent interactions that we know of, and it's probably okay to use low dose DHEA if you have diabetes. But again, physician supervision is essential.

Thyroid hormones. The combination of DHEA and thyroid hormones can lead to overstimulation, therefore, caution is indicated.

Heart medicines. DHEA is not recommended for

anyone who has a propensity for heart irregularities. If you're currently on heart medicines, be very cautious with this hormone and do not exceed 2 or 3 mg.

There are hundreds of medicines and supplements, and countless combinations. It will take us many more years to have a fuller understanding of how DHEA interacts with all of them. In the meantime, it would be a prudent idea to consult a professional health care provider whenever there is a question about the appropriateness of taking any medications in combination.

Conclusion

There is no doubt that the majority of individuals who take the appropriate dosage of DHEA notice an improvement in mood, energy, sex drive, and even an improvement in cognitive functioning, such as better memory and thinking abilities. Whether regular supplementation with DHEA for years and decades will increase life span is currently not known. My personal opinion is that we may eventually find DHEA to influence longevity in certain individuals who have low levels of this hormone. However, it will take decades to find the right dosages, the frequency, and the ideal form of administration; i.e., pills, cream, sublingual, timed-release pills, or micronized. It will also take a long time to find out which population groups would most benefit.

In the meantime, many of these hormones are easily available, and the public wants guidelines. If you plan to take these hormones, err on the side of taking less, rather than more. It's quite possible that low doses could be beneficial while high dosages could be counterproductive.

Doctors and patients are often looking for the magic pill that, by itself, will cure all ills. The human body is too complicated, with too many biochemical reactions occurring every second, for one pill to be the answer to all problems. The answer lies in intelligently combining a variety of modalities: that is, both pill and non-pill approaches.

Evaluation and supervision by a health care provider is recommended when supplementing with hormones. See www.raysahelian.com for the latest updates.

Glossary

Alzheimer's disease. A progressive brain disease leading to memory loss, interference with thinking abilities, and other losses of mental powers. Brain cells show degenerative damage.

Androgen. A hormone that encourages the development of male sexual characteristics. Some of the androgens made by the adrenal glands are DHEA, DHEAS, androstenedione, and testosterone.

Antioxidant. A substance that combines with damaging molecules, neutralizes them, and thus prevents the deterioration of DNA, RNA, lipids, and proteins. Vitamins C, E, and beta-carotene are the best known antioxidants, but more and more are being discovered each year. It is believed that one aspect of aging is the slow degeneration and breakdown of chemicals within our cells. Antioxidants are thought to prevent or slow down this degenerative process.

Cholesterol. The most abundant steroid in animal tissues. It is present in some of the foods we eat. Our liver can also make some if there's not enough in our diet.

Diosgenin. A compound found in the roots of some plants such as the yam. In the laboratory, parts of this molecule can be cleaved in order to make certain steroids. The steroid portion serves as a source from which pregnenolone, DHEA, and progesterone can be prepared. Our body is not known to have the proper enzymes to convert diosgenin into hormones. Therefore, ingesting wild yam extracts will not lead to DHEA production.

Estrogen. A hormone made by the ovaries, adrenal glands, and also in various cells of the body. Estrogen promotes female characteristics. The most common estrogens are estrone, estradiol, and estriol. Premarin, the product name of conjugated estrogens, is actually derived from the urine of horses.

Hormone. A chemical messenger produced by a gland or organ that influences a number of metabolic actions in our cells. Some hormones have been studied for a number of years, such as estrogen, which has been given to women after menopause for over 30 years.

Interleukin. similar to interferon, a small protein produced by white blood cells to fight infections and some forms of cancer. There are many types of interleukins, numbered 1, 2, 3, up to 10 or more. Some interleukins are good, others may have negative effects.

Lymphocyte. A type of white blood cell. Two major types are B lymphocytes and T lymphocytes.

Lymphokine. A substance released by lymphocytes to help with the immune function. Interferon is a type of lymphokine.

Natural killer cell. A type of white blood cell that can destroy certain cancer cells and germs.

Neuron. A brain cell. There are over 100 billion of these cells in our brain. Neurons communicate with each other through chemicals called neurotransmitters.

Neurotransmitter. A biochemical substance, such as norepinephrine, serotonin, dopamine, acetylcholine, and endorphin, that relays messages from one neuron to another.

Placebo. A dummy pill that contains no active ingredient.

Platelet. A small, round or oval cell found in the blood involved in blood clotting.

Prostate gland. A partly muscular gland surrounding the urethra at the base of the bladder. It secretes a lubricating fluid that is discharged with the sperm. Enlargement of this gland is known as BPH, benign prostatic hypertrophy.

Receptor. A special arrangement on a cell that recognizes a molecule and interacts with it. This allows the molecule to either enter the cell or stimulate it in a specific way.

Steroids. A large family of chemical substances comprising many hormones made in the adrenal gland, ovaries, testicles, and other parts of the body. Pregnenolone, DHEA, estrogen are all steroid hormones. There are also synthetic steroids manufactured by drug companies.

Testosterone. A hormone made by the testicles and adrenal glands, and also in various cells of the body, that promotes masculine traits.

References

Feldman HA, Johannes CB, McKinlay JB, Longcope C, "Low dehydroepiandrosterone sulfate and heart disease in middle-aged men: cross-sectional results from the Massachusetts Male Aging Study," *Annols of Epidemiology* (1998): 8(4):217–28.

Guazzo E, et al., "Cortisol, DHEA, and DHEAS in the CSF fluid of man: Relation to blood levels and the effecs of age," *Journal of Clinical Endocrinology and Metabolism* (1996): 81:3591–3960.

Jesse R, Loesser K, Eich D, Qian YZ, Hess ML, Nestler JE, "Dehydroepiandrosterone inhibits human platelet aggregation in vitro and in vivo," *Annals of the New York Academy of Medicine* (1995): 774:281–290.

Jones JA, Nguyen A, Straub M, Leidich RB, Veech RL, Wolf S, "Use of DHEA in a patient with advanced prostate cancer: a case report and review," *Urology* (1997): 50(5):784–788.

Khalil A, et al., "Dehydroepiandrosterone protects low density lipoproteins against peroxidation by free radicals produced by gamma-radiolysis of ethanol-water mixtures," *Atherosclerosis* (1998): 136(1):99–107.

Kimonides VG, Khatibi NH, Svendsen CN, Sofroniew MV, Herbert J, "Dehydroepiandrosterone (DHEA) and DHEA-sulfate (DHEAS) protect hippocampal neurons against excitatory amino acid-induced neurotoxicity," *Proceedings of the National Academy of Sciences* (1998): 17;95(4):1852–7.

Kurzman ID, Panciera DL, Miller JB, MacEwen EG, "The effect of dehydroepiandrosterone combined with a low-fat diet in spontaneously obese dogs: a clinical trial," *Obesity Research* (1998): 6(1):20–8.

Labrie F, Diamond P, Cusan L, Gomez JL, Belanger A, Canda B, "Effect of 12-month dehydroepiandrosterone replacement therapy on bone, vagina, and endometrium in postmenopausal women," *Journal of Clinical Endocrinology and Metabolism* (1997): 82:3498–3505.

Majewska M, "Neuronal Actions of DHEA: Possible roles in brain development, aging, memory, and affect," *Annals of the New York Academy of Sciences* (1995): 774:111–120.

Mao X, Barger SW, "Neuroprotection by dehydroepiandrosterone-sulfate: role of an NFkappaB-like factor," *Neuroreport* (1998): 9;9(4):759–63, 1998.

Orentreich N, Brind J, Rizer R, Vogelman J, "Age changes and sex differences in serum dehydroepiandrosterone sulfate concentrations throughout adulthood," *Journal of Clinical Endocrinology and Metabolism* (1984): 59:(3): 551–554.

Scheven BA, Milne JS, "Dehydroepiandrosterone (DHEA) and DHEA-S interact with 1,25-dihydroxyvitamin D3 (1,25(OH)2D3) stimulate human osteoblastic cell differentiation," *Life Sciences* (1998): 62(1):59–68.

van Vollenhoven RF, Morabito LM, Engleman EG, McGuire JL, "Treatment of systemic lupus erythematosus with dehydroepiandrosterone: 50 patients treated up to 12 months," *Journal of Rheumatology* (1998): 25(2):285–9.

Wolkowitz OM, Reus VI, Roberts E, Manfredi F, et al., "DHEA treatment of depression," *Biological Psychiatry* (1997): 41:311–18.

Yen SS, Morales AJ, Khorram O, "Replacement of DHEA in aging men and women," *Annals of the New York Academy of Sciences* (1995): 774:128–142.

Suggested Readings

Sahelian R. *DHEA: A Practical Guide*. Garden City Park, New York: Avery Publishing Group, 1996.

Sahelian R. *5-HTP: Nature's Serotonin Solution*. Garden City Park, New York: Avery Publishing Group, 1998.

Sahelian R. *Melatonin: Nature's Sleeping Pill*. Garden City Park, New York: Avery Publishing Group, 1996.

Sahelian R. *Pregnenolone: Nature's Feel Good Hormone*. Garden City Park, New York: Avery Publishing Group, 1997.

Index

Acquired immunodefi-
    ciency syndrome. *See*
    AIDS.
Aging, 12–13
  brain function and, 22–23
  DHEA and, 12–13, 18,
    19–20
  DHEA production, effect
    on, 15–16
  hormone production,
    effect on, 15–16
  physiological changes, 17
AIDS, 39–40
  DHEA and, 40–42
Aldosterone, 16
Alzheimer's disease, 23, 26
Androgens. *See* Estrogen;
    Testosterone.
Androstenedione, 12, 72
Arthritis. *See* Rheumatoid
    arthritis.
Aspirin, 72
Atherosclerosis, 30

B cells. *See* Lymphocytes.
Brain
  DHEA, aging, and, 22–33
  DHEA and cell damage
    of, 25–26
  DHEA and function of,
    21–22, 23
Breast-feeding and DHEA,
    70

Cancer, 33–36, 70
Casson, P.R., 57
CD4. *See* T cells.
Cerebrospinal fluid, 22
Cholesterol, 8, 19, 30, 54
Cortisol, 10, 16, 22, 42

Dehydroepiandrosterone.
    See DHEA.
DHA. *See* Docosahexanoic
    acid.
DHEA, 5–6
  aging and, 12–13, 15–16

AIDS and, 40–42
antidepressants, combined with, 71
antioxidant, as an, 30
behavior, effect on, 23
blood clotting and, 29
bone density and, 50–51
brain function, effect on, 21–22, 22–23, 25–26
breast-feeding and, 70
cancer and, 33–34, 36
DHEAS and, 11
dosage, suggested, 53, 56, 58–59, 61–62, 67–68
estrogen replacement and, 56–57
forms of, 55
hair and, 51, 58
heart disease and, 27–28, 30–31
HIV and, 40–42
hormones, effect upon, 11–12
immune system, effect upon, 38–39
levels of, in the body, 64–65
lupus and, 44–45
medication, taken with, 71–73
memory, effect on, 2l3, 24–25
pills, in the form of, 9. 54

pregnancy and, 52, 70
production of, in the body, 8
prostate cancer and, 34–36
rheumatoid arthritis and, 46
sex drive and, 50
side effects of, 13, 68–70
skin and, 47, 51, 68
sports, legality in using, 51
weight loss and, 49–50
what it is, 7–8
DHEA-sulfate (DHEAS), 11, 19, 28
HIV and, 41–42
rheumatoid arthritis and, 46
skin diseases and, 47
See also DHEA.
DHEAS. *See* DHEA-sulfate.
Diamond, Dr., 20
Dihydrotestosterone, 35, 36
Diosgenin, 9
Docosahexanoic acid (DHA), 7
Dyner, T.S., 41

Estrogen, 8, 12, 16, 22, 56–57, 58, 60, 71

Finasteride, 68
Flood, James, Dr., 24

Guazzo, E., 22

HDL, 19. *See also*
   Cholesterol.
Heart disease, 27
   blood thinners and,
      28–29
   DHEA as a cause of,
      30–31
   DHEA levels and, 27–28
Heart irregularities, 68
HIV, 39–40
   DHEA and, 40–42
Hormones
   production of, aging's
      effect on, 15–16
   replacement therapy,
      57–58, 58–59, 62–63
   supplements, benefits of,
      17–18
   vitamins taken with, 61
   See also Aldosterone;
      Androstenedione;
      Cortisol; DHEA;
      Dihydrotestosterone;
      Estrogen;
      Pregnenolone; Proge-
      sterone; Testosterone;
Human immunodeficiency
   virus. *See* HIV.
Immune system, 37–38

AIDS and, 39–40
   DHEA and, 38–39
Insulin, 72
Interferon, 38
Interleukin-2, 44

LDL, 19, 30. *See also*
   Cholesterol.
Lupus, 43–45
Lymphocytes, 38. *See also*
   T cells.
Lymphokines, 38

Melatonin, 16

Neurotransmitters, 21

Pemphigoid, 47
Pemphigus, 47
Pregnancy, 52, 70
Pregnenolone, 8, 57–58, 60,
   69, 72
Premarin, 60
Professional sports and
   DHEA, 51
Progesterone, 8, 57–58, 60
Propranolol, 69

RA. *See* Rheumatoid
   arthritis.
Rheumatoid arthritis (RA),
   45–46
Sports. *See* Professional
   sports.

Steroids, 8, 10, 54. *See also* DHEA.

Sterols, 9, 54

Suzuki, T., 44

Systemic lupus erythematosus (SLE). *See* Lupus.

T cells, 39–41. *See also* Lymphocytes.

Testosterone, 8, 9, 12, 35, 36, 57

Urology, 35

Van Vollenhoven, R.F., Dr., 44

Vitamin C, 30

Vitamin E, 13, 30

Vitamins
 hormones taken with, 61

Wild yam extract, 9

Wolkowitz, Owen, Dr., 23

Yam extract. *See* Wild yam extract.

Yen, Samuel, Dr., 18